KU-032-395

Contents

A new life begins

Every time a baby is born it seems like a miracle – an entirely new human being, different from everyone else, has appeared. Yet the beginning of a new life is both very ordinary and incredibly common. All around us new plants, insects and other animals are sprouting and growing. All kinds of living things must reproduce themselves if each kind is to survive. Every living thing has **organs** whose job is to create this new life.

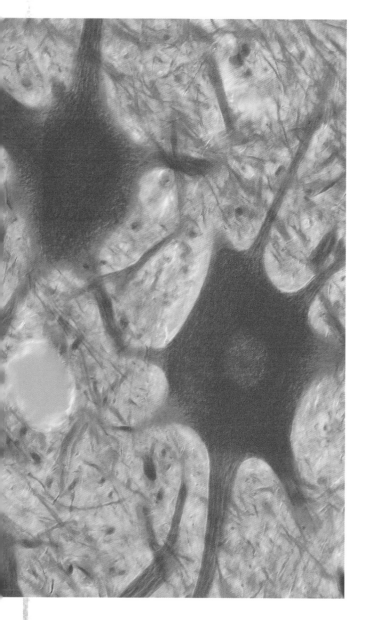

Males and females

It takes a man and a woman to make a new human life. Males and females have different sexual organs – the man's sexual organs produce male **sex cells** and the woman's produce female sex cells. A male sex cell must join with a female sex cell to make the first cell of a new person.

This first **cell** divides and multiplies to form all the different kinds of cell in the body. For nine months the growing baby develops inside the mother. By the time the baby is ready to be born the single cell has multiplied into 2000 million cells, making a new and completely separate human being!

◄ *Cells are the building blocks of all living things. This photograph shows what nerve cells in the brain look like under a microscope.*

Growing and changing

Babies go on growing and changing. At first their heads are large compared with their bodies and their arms and legs are short. As a baby becomes a child its body grows faster than its head, and its arms and legs grow faster still.

When children reach puberty, a new set of changes occurs. Their bodies become more adult and their sexual organs begin to mature and start working so that, one day, they too will be able to produce children.

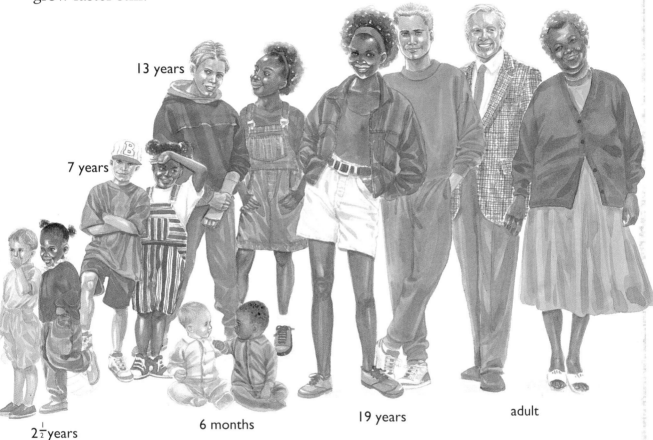

13 years

7 years

$2\frac{1}{2}$ years

6 months

19 years

adult

▲ Children not only grow bigger as they get older, they change shape too.

Did you know?

About 137 million babies are born every year – that's 258 every minute. Every kind of living thing has to reproduce to survive, but many people think that the number of humans is increasing too fast.

Growing into an adult

Puberty is the time when you start to change into an adult. Puberty usually begins some time between the ages of 11 and 14 for girls and between 13 and 16 for boys, but many people begin earlier or later. Both girls and boys grow rapidly during puberty and their bodies change shape. The sexual or reproductive **organs** begin to work. These changes are brought about by **hormones**, which affect the emotions too.

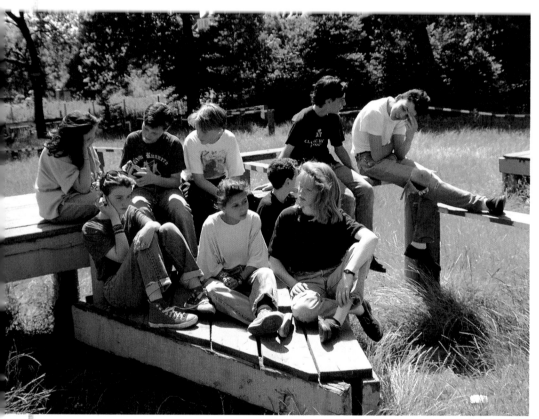

◀ Teenagers often spend hours sitting around and talking. Their emotions and interests are developing as well as their bodies.

Physical changes

During puberty a girl's breasts begin to grow, her waist becomes smaller and her hips wider. Her **ovaries** start to release eggs and her **periods** begin. A boy's shoulders and chest broaden. His **penis** becomes thicker and longer and his **testicles** produce **sperm**.

For both girls and boys, hair begins to grow more thickly on some parts of the body, particularly between the legs and under the arms. Girls also notice hair growing on their legs, and boys notice it on their faces and on their chests.

A boy's voice becomes much deeper and 'breaks'. His **vocal cords**, which produce the sound, grow so quickly that the **muscles** which control them may sometimes become confused. His voice may wobble uncontrollably between high and low until the muscles find the right tension.

Changing attitudes

Puberty doesn't only bring changes in the body. It also affects emotions and attitudes. Teenagers become acutely aware of how they look and may become sexually attracted to members of the opposite sex. They slowly become more independent and responsible for themselves and others.

Parents and teenagers often argue about how independent they are ready to be! Some teenagers feel they can only assert their independence by being rebellious.

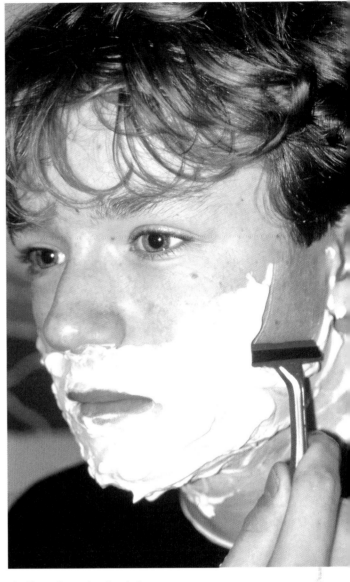

▲ For a boy, shaving is just one of the changes of puberty.

Did you know?

Girls have just as many body hairs as boys, even on their faces. As boys grow older their body hair just becomes thicker, longer and more noticeable. Probably the longest beard of all was grown by a Norwegian, Hans Langseth. When he died in 1927 it was over 5.3m long.

The woman's body

The female sex **organs** are mainly hidden inside the body. They have two main purposes – to produce eggs and provide a safe place (the **womb**) for the baby to develop. The eggs are stored in the **ovaries**, which are linked to the womb by the two thin **Fallopian tubes**. The womb is connected to the outside of the body by the **cervix** and **vagina**. The opening to the vagina is in the folds of skin between the legs.

An egg is released

Every month the female **reproductive system** gets ready to make a new baby. An egg matures in one of the ovaries and is released into the Fallopian tube. An egg will live only for 12 to 24 hours unless it is **fertilized** in the tube by a **sperm**. As the egg travels down the tube, the lining of the womb becomes thicker. It is ready for a fertilized egg to embed itself. If the egg has not been fertilized, it dies and does not embed itself.

Periods

The unwanted lining and egg are then washed out of the womb in a slow flow of blood through the vagina. The flow of blood is called **menstruation**, or more simply a **period**. It usually lasts about five days to a week, and there may be some pain at the beginning. Women wear pads or insert a **tampon** into the vagina to absorb the blood. Both pads and tampons have to be changed every few hours. At the end of the period, the whole cycle begins again.

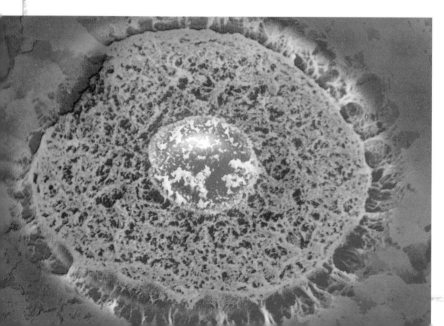

◄ *An egg (the green ball) erupting from the ovary to begin its journey down the Fallopian tube. The photo has been coloured to show the egg more clearly.*

The first period

Girls are born with all the eggs already formed in their ovaries. But the eggs do not start to mature and a girl's sexual organs do not start working until around her early teens. At first her periods may occur fairly haphazardly, but as her body gets used to the monthly cycle, her periods become more regular.

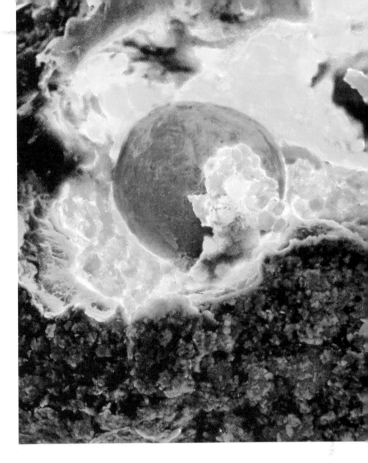

► This photo shows an egg (red ball in the centre) entering the Fallopian tube. It is magnified about 2000 times.

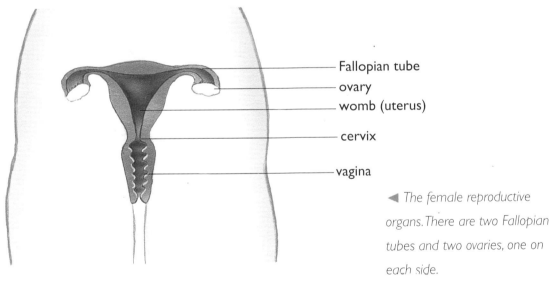

Fallopian tube
ovary
womb (uterus)
cervix
vagina

◄ The female reproductive organs. There are two Fallopian tubes and two ovaries, one on each side.

Did you know?

A baby girl is born with about 300,000 eggs in her ovaries. By the time she is 12 years old only about 10,000 are still capable of being fertilized. Of these just over 400 will be released one by one until the ovaries stop releasing eggs, usually when the woman is about 50.

The man's body

A man's sex **organs** are easier to see than a woman's. They have two purposes – to make **sperm** (the male **sex cells**) and to place them inside the woman's body. Sperm are made and stored in the two **testicles** contained in a pouch, called the scrotum, behind the **penis**. Sperm leave the man's body through the penis.

A long journey

The testicles hang outside the body to keep them cool – if sperm become too warm they die. Sperm travel to the penis through a long tube called the **vas deferens**. On the way they become mixed with a fluid called semen. When a man is sexually excited, his penis fills with blood and becomes stiff. Rapid contractions of the **muscles** at the base of the penis cause the semen and sperm to spurt, or ejaculate, from the tip of the penis.

During puberty a boy's penis may become stiff (or erect) and ejaculate sperm while he is asleep. This is called a 'wet dream'.

The penis

As well as ejaculating sperm and semen, the penis empties **urine** from the **bladder**. There is no danger of these two functions getting mixed up. When the penis becomes stiff, the tube from the bladder is blocked off.

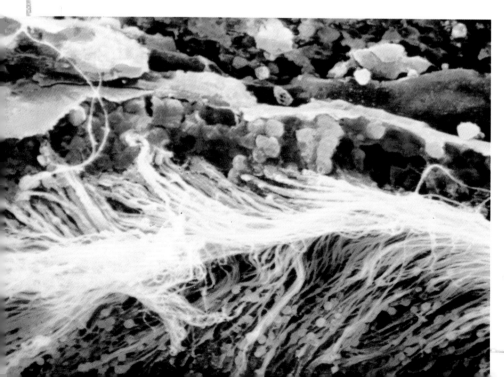

◀ This photo has been colour tinted. The fine purple strands are the tails of sperm being made in a tiny tube in the testicle. The sperm are then stored in the **epididymis** alongside the testicle.

Foreskin

The tip of the penis is protected by a fold of skin called the **foreskin**. When the penis becomes erect, the foreskin slides back. Some boys have their foreskin removed soon after birth in an operation known as circumcision. This is usually for religious reasons, or because it is then easier to keep clean.

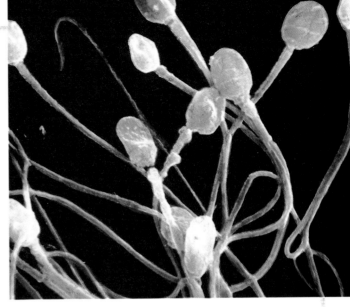

▲ *A sperm looks a bit like a tadpole. The head carries the sex cell and the long tail thrashes to and fro to move the sperm along.*

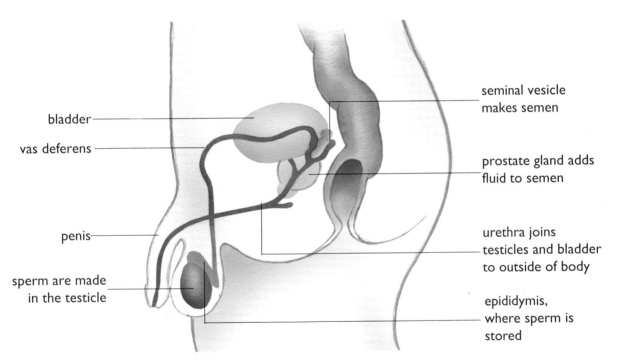

seminal vesicle makes semen

bladder

vas deferens

prostate gland adds fluid to semen

penis

urethra joins testicles and bladder to outside of body

sperm are made in the testicle

epididymis, where sperm is stored

▲ *The male reproductive organs.*

Did you know?

Sperm are tiny. About 20 laid head to tail would measure only 1mm. After puberty the testicles make about 200 million sperm every day. They can survive for several weeks in the epididymis before they die and turn to liquid.

Joining together

Conception, the start of a new life, occurs when a man's **sperm** joins with a woman's egg as it travels down one of her **Fallopian tubes**. So how does the sperm get to the unfertilized egg? The answer is by **sexual intercourse**, which is often simply called 'sex' or 'making love'. The man puts his **penis** inside the woman's **vagina** and ejaculates sperm. The sperm then race to reach the egg.

Making love

When a couple become sexually aroused the man's penis becomes stiff and erect and the woman's vagina becomes wet and slippery. This makes it easy for his penis to be inserted into her vagina. They move his penis back and forwards in the vagina, until the man ejaculates and semen and sperm spurt into her.

The sperm race

Sperm use their long tails to swim up the vagina and into the womb. About 500 million sperm start the race at high speed. These tiny **cells** have to swim upstream and have just a few hours to reach the egg. Only a few hundred reach the Fallopian tube and only one of these can **fertilize** the egg.

Did you know?

Once inside the vagina, sperm have to travel about 15–18 cm to reach the egg. This may not sound far, but remember that sperm are only $\frac{1}{20}$ mm long, so the equivalent for you would be swimming 5 km.

◄ The moment of fertilization. The sperm (blue) has just broken through the egg's cell wall (pink). Its long tail stays outside – only the head joins with the egg.

The egg is surrounded by layers of cells. Sperm try to fight their way in. At last one sperm breaks through the cell **membrane** which then thickens so that no other sperm can enter. The egg has now been fertilized, and a new life has begun.

Close and loving

Sexual intercourse is not just a biological necessity. It is the closest way for a couple to share their love. Having sex does not always lead to conception. **Contraception** helps to make sure it doesn't.

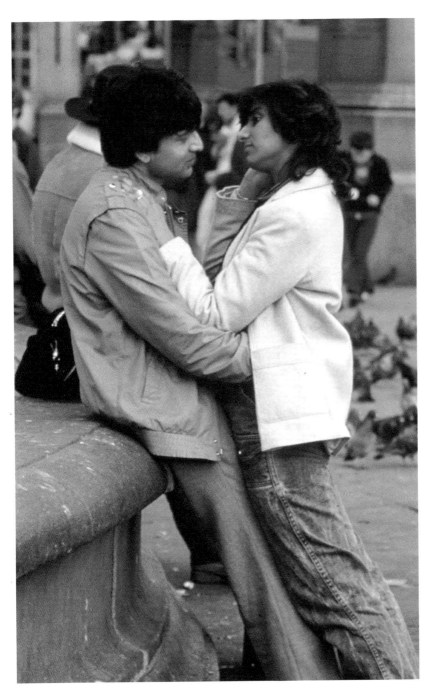

◄ A couple can express love for each other in many ways. They can show their love by speaking and listening to each other, sharing what they have, helping each other and enjoying doing things together, as well as through hugs and kisses!

The first hours

As soon as a **sperm** joins with the egg, something amazing happens. The new **cell** begins to copy itself and a few hours later it splits into two cells. Every 12 hours the number of cells doubles so that the two cells become four cells, then eight, and so on. By the time it reaches the **womb** it has become a ball of about 64 cells. If the cluster of cells is to survive it must implant itself in the lining of the womb. There the cells continue to divide. They form different kinds of cells and organize themselves into the **embryo** of a new human being.

Blueprint for life

How can different kinds of cell form from just one cell? The answer lies in **chromosomes**. Chromosomes carry a set of coded instructions which tell each kind of cell what to do and how to reproduce itself. The **nucleus** of the egg and sperm each contain a half set of chromosomes which join together to make a new combination of chromosomes. Before a cell divides it copies the chromosomes so that each new cell has full identical set.

◀ *This magnified and artificially coloured photo shows a cluster of cells four days after the egg was **fertilized** and just before it implants itself in the wall of the womb.*

A question of looks

As well as telling each kind of cell what to do, chromosomes decide exactly how you will look – the colour of your eyes, the shape of your nose, and so on. They also decide which sex you will be.

Since you have inherited half your chromosomes from your mother and half from your father, you will share some characteristics with each of them. You may not think that you look very like your parents or brothers and sisters, but no doubt other people say you do. It's incredible to think that the way you look now was determined from the moment the first cell formed.

▼ Before a cell divides, it copies the chromosomes to form two complete sets. The cell then divides into two so that each cell has an identical set of chromosomes.

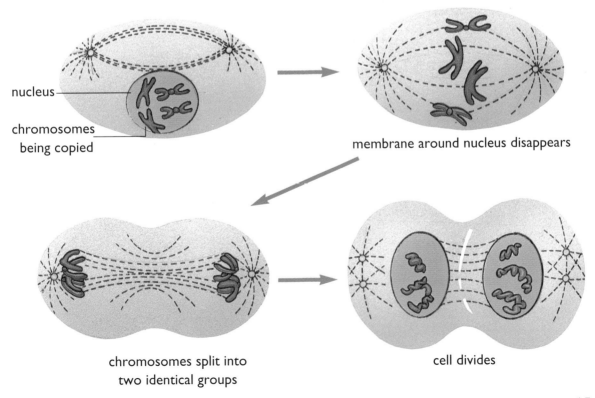

nucleus

chromosomes being copied

membrane around nucleus disappears

chromosomes split into two identical groups

cell divides

The first eight weeks

In the first eight weeks of life the human **embryo** changes from a cluster of **cells** to the recognizable shape of a human being. It spends its time in the **womb** floating in a bag of liquid. It doesn't need to breathe or eat, because all the oxygen and food it needs until it is born comes from the mother.

The growing embryo

Three weeks after **conception**, the embryo is about the size of a grain of rice but already cells have developed which will form all the different parts of the body – blood, **muscles**, bones, skin, hair and internal **organs**.

A week later the embryo has doubled in size. It is now 7 mm long and its tiny heart has begun to beat.

At six weeks the embryo is just over 1 cm long. Its stomach, liver and kidneys have formed and its head is beginning to develop. Its arms and legs are tiny buds. Two weeks later, at eight weeks, the eyes, ears and even tiny fingers are forming, yet the embryo is still only 4 cm long – smaller than your little finger.

▼ *This embryo is four weeks old. The head and spine are beginning to form. The red bulge is the heart.*

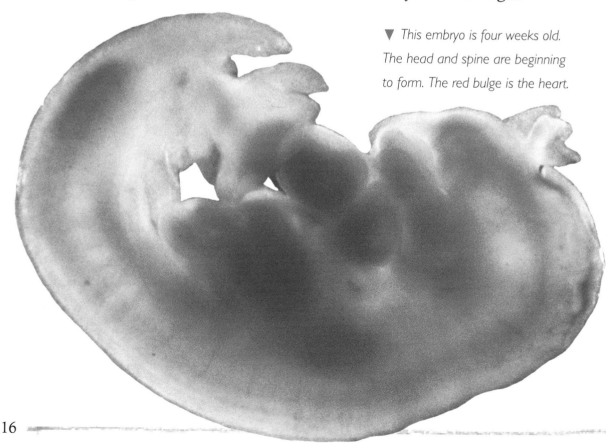

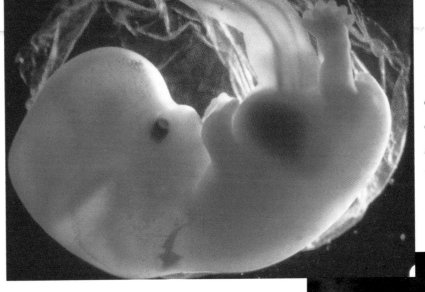

◄ The embryo seven weeks after conception. The eyes are already forming. The head is huge compared to the body.

Capsule for survival

Only a few of the 64 cells that first reached the womb grow into the baby itself. Most form the **placenta** and a protective skin, or **membrane**, which makes a bag around the embryo and fills with **amniotic fluid**. The embryo floats in this liquid, protected from bumps and bangs. The placenta is a spongy lump connected to the embryo by the **umbilical cord**. The placenta allows food and oxygen from the mother's blood to pass along the cord to the growing embryo. It also takes waste away from the embryo's blood.

Did you know?

The lungs begin to form when the embryo is just 7 weeks old, but it does not use them to breathe while it is in the womb. The lungs develop slowly and are filled with a salty liquid. While the baby is in the womb, it gets all the oxygen it needs from the mother's blood. When the baby is born, the lungs have to pump away the fluid quickly and get ready to take in air.

▲ This baby is almost ready to be born. You can get an idea of its size by comparing its backbone with that of the mother.

Growing bigger

At eight weeks the **embryo** is almost human-shaped, and from now on it is called a **fetus**. By the end of 14 weeks the body is fully formed, but it will spend another 24 weeks in the **womb**. In that time the baby will grow bigger and its **organs** will mature so that it can survive after birth outside the womb. As it gets bigger, the mother's womb stretches to make room for it and she becomes more and more aware of the baby moving inside her.

The first kick

At 14 weeks the **muscles** are beginning to grow and, as they get stronger, the fetus moves its arms and legs more vigorously. But it is only 12 cm long. It may be another six weeks before its mother can feel its feet kicking against her belly.

By then the fetus has doubled in size and the mother's womb is beginning to bulge. By six months the fetus would probably survive if it were born, although only if it were looked after in the protected environment of an **incubator**.

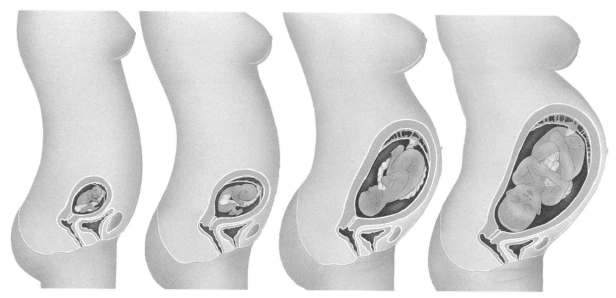

at 10 weeks fetus weighs about 18 g

at 14 weeks fetus weighs about 135 g

at 24 weeks fetus weighs about 700 g

at 36 weeks fetus weighs about 3.4 kg

▲ An unborn baby grows more quickly than at any other time in life. The mother's womb stretches as the baby grows.

Life inside the womb

For the final three months in the womb, the fetus continues to grow stronger and put on weight. It becomes more aware of its surroundings. It sucks its thumb and can hear its mother's heart beating. It will even jump if there is a loud noise. From about 20 weeks the fetus sleeps and can open and shut its eyes.

Its mother becomes increasingly aware of it. Towards the end of **pregnancy** she can feel its arms and legs moving and she can feel it hiccupping! All this time the fetus is supplied with food and oxygen from her blood through the **placenta**. By about the 38th week, the placenta begins to fail and the baby is ready to be born.

► This pregnant woman is having an **ultrasound** scan. She can watch her unborn baby moving inside her as the doctors check that the fetus is well and healthy. The machine uses sound echoes to build up the picture.

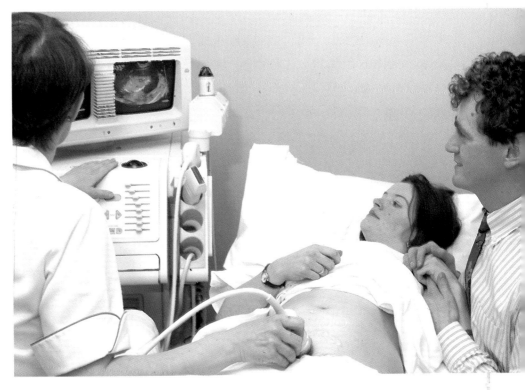

Did you know?

Anything in the mother's blood can pass to her unborn baby through the placenta, including the poisons of cigarettes and drugs. When a mother smokes, her baby is deprived of vital oxygen. This can affect its mental and physical development. Unborn babies can even become addicted to drugs.

Giving birth

A mother becomes increasingly heavy and uncomfortable towards the end of the **pregnancy**. She can't wait for the baby to be born. Giving birth is called labour and it is hard work for the mother. The **womb**, which is largely made of **muscle**, contracts to push the baby out. But first the **cervix** has to stretch to allow the baby through into the **vagina**.

First signs

A week or two before labour, the baby usually turns in the womb so that its head is facing down towards the cervix. Often the first sign of labour is increasing spasms of pain in the belly, rather like **period** pains.

The pains are caused by the cervix slowly stretching. It can take 10, 12 or even 18 hours for the cervix to open fully to a diameter of 10 cm, and during that time the pain becomes more and more intense.

▶ This baby is ready to be born. The cervix, which is still tightly closed, will stretch and open to allow the baby's head through.

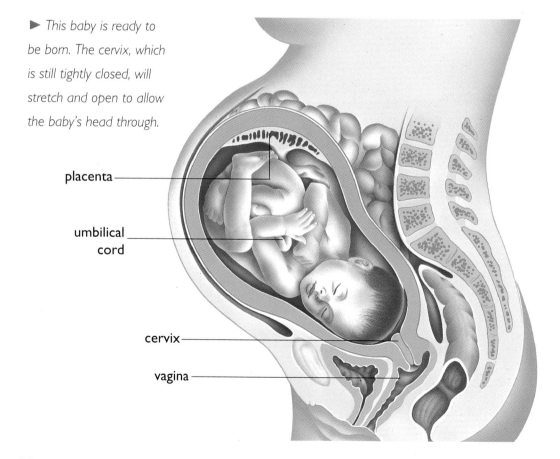

placenta

umbilical cord

cervix

vagina

Painkillers

Most women prepare for childbirth and practise breathing and relaxation exercises to help them cope with the pain. If the pain is too great, however, there are different kinds of painkiller to help them. They are given by the midwives or doctors.

Pushing the baby out

When the cervix is fully open, the muscular walls of the womb begin to contract. Slowly the baby is pushed through the cervix and into the vagina, which stretches easily to let the baby through. The mother helps by pushing hard as the womb contracts. This stage of childbirth is shorter – usually an hour or less. Once the baby's head has emerged the rest of the body follows easily. The baby has been born! The birth, however, is not over until the **placenta** has been pushed out too.

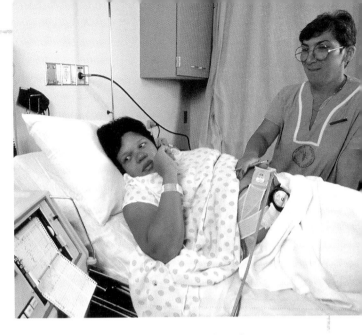

▲ A machine **monitors** the baby's heartbeat as labour progresses.

Did you know?

Many babies and mothers used to die from infections and complications. Today's midwives and doctors monitor the baby and mother and take action if problems arise. Some babies are born by **Caesarean** section. A cut is made into the womb and the baby is lifted out.

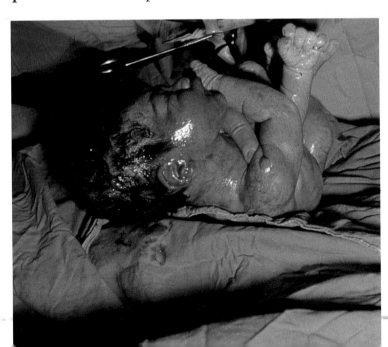

◄ This baby has just been born. The **umbilical cord** is still attached to his mother.

A newborn baby

It must be a big shock to a baby to leave the warmth and comfort of the **womb** and find itself in the world outside. It is almost totally helpless and must rely on others to look after it, but it is equipped with several **instincts** and **reflexes**. Some of these help it survive but others seem irrelevant and do not last long. Don't try to test any of these reactions – they can disappear at any time. Newborn babies must always be handled very carefully.

The first cry

As soon as the baby is born something amazing happens. It opens its mouth, takes a gasp of air, splutters, coughs and cries! Up until now the lungs and breathing tubes have been full of fluid. Now the lungs no longer make fluid.

Instead, they absorb it and get ready to take in oxygen from the air instead. As soon as the baby has started breathing, the midwife or doctor clamps the **umbilical cord** and cuts it. The baby is now surviving on his or her own for the first time.

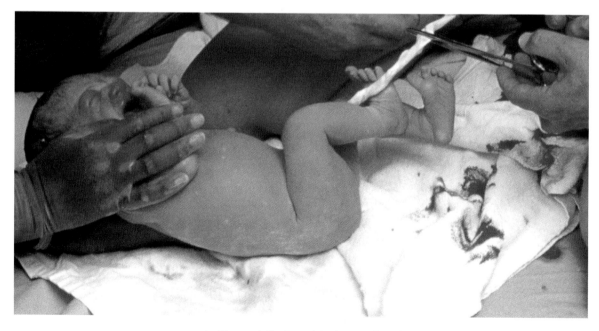

▲ *The umbilical cord is clamped and cut. It must be kept very clean until it shrivels and falls off naturally about a week after birth.*

The first feed

Both the mother and baby are ready for breast-feeding. The baby has a strong instinct to suck and will feed from the mother's breast. During **pregnancy** the breasts become larger and get ready to produce milk. As soon as the baby begins to suck, a cloudy, nutritious liquid called **colostrum** begins to flow. Within a few days it is followed by milk.

Reflexes

A reflex is something you do without thinking. If something touches your eyelashes, you automatically blink. Newborn babies blink, sneeze and swallow automatically. They also have several reflexes which don't last more than a week or two. For example, if you put a finger in each of its palms it will grip so tightly you can pick the baby up.

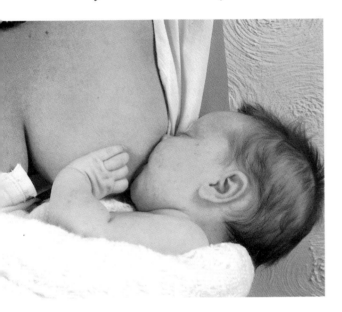

◄ Babies suck automatically. Breast milk has all the nourishment they need. A baby also loves the warm comfort of a cuddle.

Did you know?

All babies are born with blue eyes. They may change to brown within a few hours but sometimes it takes longer – several days or weeks. Some babies are born with hair on their heads, others are bald. A few are even born with a tooth.

▼ A newborn baby's tiny fingers can grip surprisingly tightly.

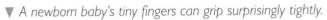
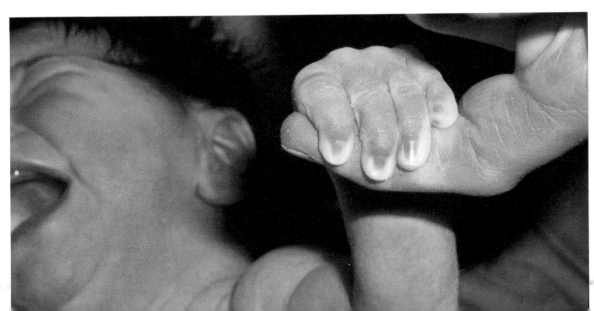

More about chromosomes

Everything about the way you look and even whether you are a girl or boy was decided by the **chromosomes** which you inherited from your parents. Chromosomes are made up of **genes** and they carry coded information which tell the **cells** how to grow. The code includes which sex you are, the colour of your hair and eyes, and the shape of your body.

A boy or a girl?

Body cells contain 46 chromosomes, but **sex cells** (eggs and **sperm**) have only 23 each. When an egg and sperm join, the new cell has 46 chromosomes. There are 22 matching pairs and one pair which sometimes matches and sometimes not. This pair carries the coded information which makes you a boy or a girl.

Girls always have two matching chromosomes shaped like an X, but boys have one X chromosome and one chromosome which is shaped more like a Y. While all female eggs carry an X chromosome, some sperm carry a Y chromosome and some an X chromosome. So the sex of a child is decided by the father's sperm.

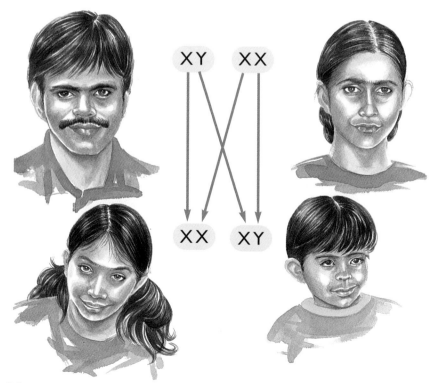

◄ Follow the arrows to see how a boy inherits an X chromosome from his mother and a Y chromosome from his father. Girls always inherit and pass on X chromosomes.

Dominant features

Chromosomes contain two instructions for every characteristic, one from each parent. Sometimes both instructions work together, but sometimes one instruction overrules the other. If you inherit a gene for brown eyes and a gene for blue eyes, your eyes will be brown. Similarly brown hair always predominates over fair hair. However if both parents have brown eyes, but carry a 'hidden gene' for blue eyes and their child inherits this gene from both of them, he or she will have blue eyes.

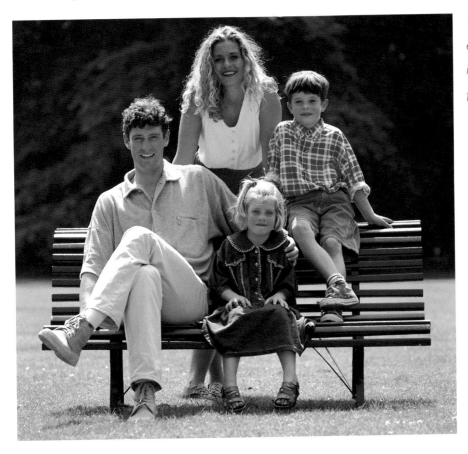

◄ Can you see what each child has inherited from the parents?

Did you know?

Henry VIII of England was determined to have a son to succeed him as King of England, but his wives kept giving birth to girls. He divorced two wives and executed two because they had not 'given' him a son. If only those wives could have told him it was he who had failed to produce a cell with a Y chromosome – so it was his problem all along!

Twins and triplets

Twins are two babies who grow in the **womb** at the same time and are born within a few hours or days of each other. It can be quite confusing to meet two people who look exactly the same – which one is which? But not all twins look alike, because twins are formed in two different ways, producing identical or dissimilar twins.

Identical twins

Chromosomes are inherited coded instructions that make sure each one of us is different from anyone else. If a single egg or cluster of eggs splits soon after **fertilization**, the resulting two **embryos** have identical chromosomes. This means that the twins must be of the same sex and will look alike. However, even identical twins are not exactly the same and their families can always tell them apart.

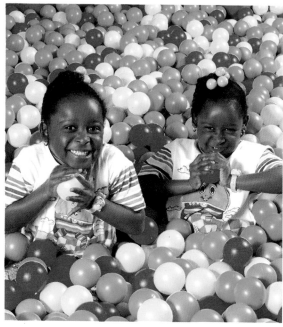

▲ *Some identical twins like to emphasize the things they have in common and dress the same.*

◄ *Others prefer to see themselves as separate individuals.*

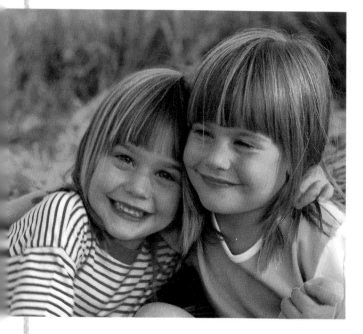

Identical twins do have a lot in common, though. They often have the same mannerisms and like and dislike the same things. Some twins claim that they know what the other twin is thinking, and that they feel pain when the other is hurt.

Did you know?

Most mothers have one, two or three children, but in the late 1700s a Russian peasant, Madame Vassilyev, gave birth to 69 babies! She had four sets of quadruplets, seven sets of triplets and 16 pairs of twins.

Dissimilar twins

Usually only one egg is released from one of the **ovaries** when a woman **ovulates**, but sometimes she may release two eggs in the same month. If both eggs are fertilized, then she will give birth to dissimilar twins. Dissimilar twins do not have the same chromosomes.

They are no more alike than any other brothers and sisters. They can be a girl and a boy or the same sex. Twins occur about once in every 90,000 **pregnancies** and they tend to run in families. So if there are twins in your family, you are more likely to have twins yourself.

▼ *These **sextuplets** include two sets of identical twins. Can you spot them?*

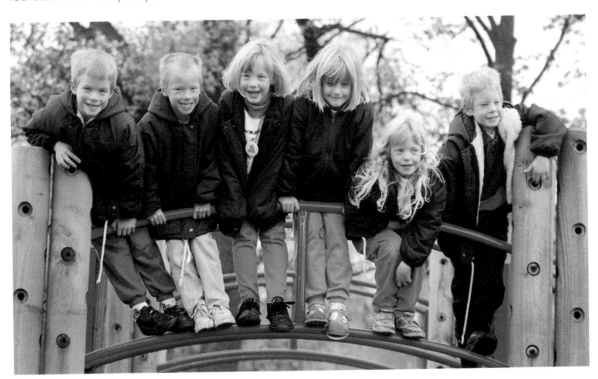

Safe sex

Sex is a pleasurable experience and a way for two people to share their love, but there are risks. To begin with, how can they make sure they don't conceive a baby by mistake? The answer is **contraception**. Another risk is catching a **sexually transmitted disease (STD)**. This is a disease which is spread by **sexual intercourse**. If a couple do have sex, the safest precaution against these risks is to use a condom.

Contraception

A condom is a rubber sheath which is rolled down over the man's erect **penis**. The **sperm** spurt into the space at the end and do not come into contact with the **vagina**. It is one of the oldest methods of contraception and, if it is used properly, it is reliable. Other methods include the pill, chemical creams, the coil, and a diaphragm, but none of them protect against sexually transmitted diseases (STDs).

Sexually transmitted diseases

There are several diseases which are passed on through unprotected sexual intercourse. The two most common cause an uncomfortable itch or genital warts. They can be treated easily if they are caught early enough. The most serious STD is **AIDS** (acquired immuno-deficiency syndrome). The human immuno-deficiency virus (**HIV**), which causes AIDS, lives in blood, semen and other body fluids.

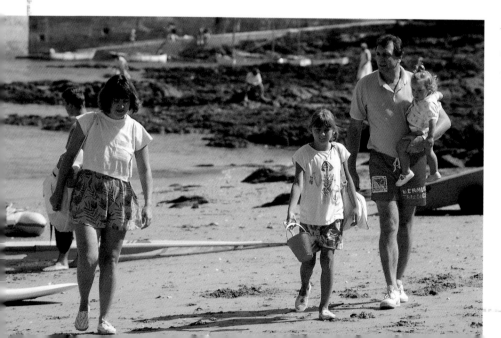

◄ *This couple use contraception except when they want to have a child.*

The HIV virus has to enter the body directly into the blood or body fluid. It is most likely to do so during unprotected sex, or when drug users share needles.

Within a few years of infection with HIV, a person usually develops AIDS, a disease in which the body's own ability to fight infection has been wrecked.

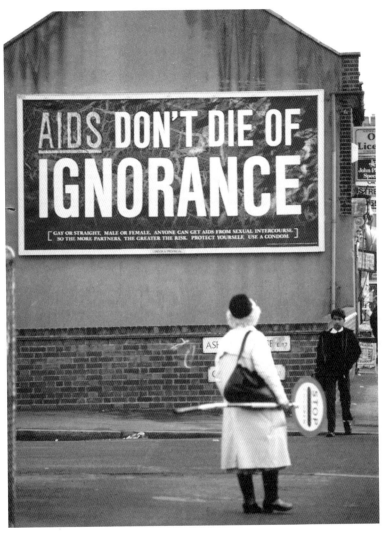

◀ When HIV was first identified in the 1980s, this poster warned people of the danger of catching AIDS from unprotected sex, and reminded them to use a condom. Look around you and you will see that new posters are produced all the time to carry this important message.

Did you know?

Even thousands of years ago people were trying to find ways of preventing unwanted pregnancies. In Ancient Egypt women used to put honey in the vagina. Roman men made condoms from the thick, stretchy bladders of animals, but they wore them mainly to protect themselves against sexually transmitted diseases.

Glossary

Abdomen The part of the body we sometimes call the 'tummy'. It includes the stomach, liver and other organs, including the sexual organs.

Addicted Having a craving for something, such as cigarettes or drugs. Some substances are **addictive**. After taking them for some time, the body cannot do without them.

AIDS Acquired immuno-deficiency syndrome – a disease in which the body's ability to fight other diseases has been damaged.

Amniotic fluid Liquid which surrounds the developing embryo and fetus in the womb and protects it from bumps and bangs.

Bladder Part of the body where urine is stored before being excreted from the body.

Caesarean section An operation in which the muscular wall of the womb is cut and the baby removed.

Cell This is the smallest living unit. Each part of the body is made of a different kind of cell.

Cervix The lower end, or neck, of the womb. It joins the womb to the vagina.

Chromosomes Tiny strands of chemicals found in the nucleus of each cell. They carry the coded instructions which tell the cells what to do. Chromosomes are inherited from the parents in the sex cells and make every individual unique.

Colostrum Cloudy liquid formed in a mother's breast in the first few days of breast-feeding.

Conception The moment at which a female egg and a sperm join together to produce the first cell of a new individual.

Contraception A way of preventing conception, for example, by using a condom during sexual intercourse.

Embryo A developing baby from the first division of cells until all the main structures have formed. In humans this is eight weeks after conception.

Epididymis Part of the testicle where sperm is stored.

Fallopian tubes Narrow tubes which carry eggs from the ovaries to the womb.

Fertilization The joining together of a female sex cell and a male sex cell. A female egg (sex cell) must be fertilized before it can grow into a new individual.

Fetus The unborn baby from eight weeks after conception until birth.

Foreskin A fold of skin which covers the tip of the penis.

Genes Parts of the chromosomes. They carry the code for inherited characteristics.

HIV (human immuno-deficiency virus) Virus which attacks the capacity of the body to defend itself against infection.

Hormones Chemicals produced by the body to control various processes. Sex hormones control the release of the eggs from a woman's ovaries and the production of sperm in a man's testicles. Female sex hormones also control the changes in a woman's body during pregnancy and birth.

Incubator A special cot for babies who are born too early. The incubator keeps the baby at a constant temperature and monitors its breathing and heartbeat.

Instinct Behaviour which is present at birth – it does not have to be learned.

Membrane A thin layer around each cell which allows food and oxygen to enter the cell and waste to leave it.

Menstruation The process by which, once a month, the lining of the womb and the unfertilized egg leave the woman's body in a slow flow of blood.

Monitor Keep a continuous record so that problems can be detected immediately.

Muscle bundles of fibres which contract (shorten) to produce movement.

Nucleus The central part of a cell which contains chromosomes and so controls what the cell does.

Organ A part of the body which does a particular job. The purpose of the sexual organs is to create new life.

Ovary The part of a woman's body where the sex cells (eggs) are stored and where some female sex hormones are made. There are two ovaries.

Ovulate To release an egg from one of the ovaries. After puberty a woman ovulates about once a month until she is about 50 years old. Ovulation stops during pregnancy.

Placenta An organ made from womb cells and by the embryo which allows food and oxygen to pass from the mother to the developing baby without their blood coming into contact. It also takes waste from the baby's blood to the mother's blood.

Penis The part of a man's body through which sperm and urine leave the body.

Period See **Menstruation.**

Pregnancy The time during which a woman carries an unborn baby in her womb. Her body goes through various changes to accommodate the growing embryo and fetus.

Reflex Automatic reactions which you do without thinking.

Reproductive system All the parts of the body which are used for reproduction (creating a new life).

Sex cell Sex cells are produced by the sexual organs to create new life. A woman's sex cells are tiny eggs produced in the ovaries. A man's sex cells are sperm produced in the testicles.

Sextuplets Six babies which develop in the womb at the same time and are born within hours of each other.

Sexual intercourse The process in which a man's erect penis is put into a women's vagina and sperm are released.

Sperm Male sex cells.

STD (sexually transmitted disease) A disease which is passed from one person to another during sexual intercourse.

Tampon A cylinder of absorbent material which is placed in the vagina to soak up the blood during menstruation.

Testicle The part of a man's body where the sex cells are manufactured and stored and male sex hormones are made. A man has two testicles.

Ultrasound A process which gives a picture of an unborn baby inside the womb using sounds and their echoes.

Umbilical cord The tube which carries blood vessels which connect the developing baby to the placenta. After birth the cord is cut and it shrivels to form the navel, or belly-button.

Urine Fluid containing waste material from the blood mixed with water.

Vagina The tube that leads from the cervix and womb to the outside of a woman's body.

Vas deferens A long, thin tube which connects the testicles to the penis.

Vocal cords Two bands of tough tissue in the throat which vibrate as you breathe out to produce sound.

Womb The part of a woman's body where a fertilized egg develops into a baby.

Index